Fruit Detox

Learn how to do an easy fruit detox cleanse, lose weight, and feel better fast!

Copyright 2015

Table Of Contents

Introduction 1

Chapter 1: The Basics and Top Benefits of Fruit Detox 2

Chapter 2: Best Foods for Detox 5

Chapter 3: How to Get Started with and Follow the Program
.... 10

Chapter 4: Juicing Guidelines on Fruit Detox Diet 16

Chapter 5: What to Expect on a Fruit Detox Diet 20

Conclusion 23

Introduction

I want to thank you and congratulate you for downloading the book, "Fruit Detox".

This book contains helpful information about detoxing, and all of its benefits!

Due to our lifestyle choices, and food habits, many people's organs are not running at their optimum levels. The organ most effected is the liver, which is responsible for breaking down toxins in the body.

During a detox, the liver gets a much needed break and is able to remove all unwanted toxins from the body. This results in our organs running better, our metabolism improving, and also gives us more energy!

This book will teach you how to do a simple fruit detox that will help you achieve all of these benefits and more!

The simple 3 to 4 day detox plan outlined in this book is a great way to cleanse your system and kick-start weight loss.

You will discover exactly how a detox works, and why they are so important to do from time to time.

So read on, and feel better fast with the fruit detox method!

Thanks again for downloading this book, I hope you enjoy it!

Chapter 1:
The Basics and Top Benefits of Fruit Detox

We get exposed to toxic materials every day. They come from the environment, and more so from the foods we eat. When toxins build up in the body, it gets much harder to flush out. The liver, which is mainly responsible for natural detox, has a tougher time eliminating these waste products.

With a cleansing diet, particularly a fruit detox, the unhealthy materials and fats can be eliminated from the body. The cleansing diet can effectively come to the rescue of the liver so that it can fulfill its role in metabolism. As your metabolism is improved through cleansing the body, you are more likely to lose weight.

It then makes sense to relieve the liver first from its toxic burden. This way, you are able to free up sufficient space in order to burn fat. And such a result can be achieved through fruit cleansing.

What is Fruit Detox?

Fruit detox is basically using the natural cleansing properties of fruits to aid in weight loss, increase stamina and improve overall health. The three day fruit cleanse in particular came from a nutritionist and fitness trainer named Jay Robb. The main purpose of fruit detox as the name itself suggests, is detoxification.

For three days, dieters have to follow a very specific meal plan consisting mainly of fruits, vegetables and protein shakes.

What are the Benefits of this Detox Program?

Many detox programs do not feature a source of protein. The inclusion of protein in this detox program is quite helpful. It works to prevent the loss of muscle mass while ensuring the elimination of toxins from the body.

It helps you lose weight.

The liver plays a major role in the breakdown of fat. As a matter of fact, the liver is as important as the stomach and the intestines. The liver is capable of producing bile and the bile assists in digesting fats. As the role of the liver and its health is improved through the cleansing diet, it is capable of helping further with the metabolism of fats. So, if you want to lose weight, you will definitely benefit from this diet.

Another great reason why you should consider this cleanse, is to eliminate liver stones that can possibly build up. This can develop as a result of excess amounts of cholesterol. This is what makes the bile develop into hard and crystalline stones. These stones can become an impediment inside the liver and may affect the gall bladder as well.

With the presence of stones as blockage, the liver may become less able to help with the natural detoxification process occurring within the body. The liver stones also stop the organ from ensuring proper distribution and delivery of nutrients throughout the body. Moreover, an imbalance may be experienced particularly affecting the proper retention of water and salt.

It cleanses the body.

Because the liver is one of the body parts with a big role to play in the detoxification process, it is essential that you exert effort in giving it the help it needs. It is the responsibility of the liver to convert toxic substances into harmless elements. Such occurs in the two phases of the detox process.

There are instances when not all of the toxins in the liver are properly eliminated. This problem may arise if the liver becomes compromised. However, with the help of the cleansing diet, these foreign elements can be completely eliminated and this helps to restore the liver to normal, allowing it to perform at optimum levels.

It provides an energy boost.

The liver is capable of converting one substance into a different form. This means as toxins enter the liver, they get synthesized into less harmful elements and most of them get excreted as waste. There are some elements that are converted into other forms which the body may actually use to function. The problem is when the liver is not in good shape, it may not be able to release the nutrients back into the body through the bloodstream.

With the help of a fruit cleanse, the supply of nutrients can be restored. And such can help give you a boost of energy which can be useful in allowing you to perform your daily activities, including exercise.

Chapter 2:
Best Foods for Detox

If you want to cleanse your system, get healthy and lose weight in the process, you should be looking for the most helpful foods for your detox. Some of the best foods include the following:

Apple

Apples are rich in pectin. Pectin cleanses, and allows the body to release harmful toxins from the digestive tract. Because of this pectin content in apples, it makes it much easier for the liver to manage the toxic burden in the process of cleansing.

You can eat apples whole and raw. You may also juice this fruit. For variety, you may make an unsweetened apple sauce or serve apples slices with almond butter. You can also have a bowl of apple slices with berries, almonds, flaxseeds and a sprinkle of cinnamon for breakfast or snacks.

Avocado

This is another antioxidant rich fruit. It has the ability to reduce cholesterol levels and dilate the blood vessels. This fruit also has carcinogen blocking ability thanks to its glutathione content, and is able to block 30 different carcinogens. At the same time, this nutrient in avocado assists the liver in eliminating synthetic chemicals from the body.

You can enjoy avocado by adding it to a smoothie recipe, or by making it in to a tasty and creamy dip.

Blueberries

Rich in the phytonutrient proanthocyanidins, blueberries have a super detoxifying ability. In addition, this fruit also contains antiviral and anti inflammation properties. If you take 300 grams of blueberries, you can be assured of protection from DNA damage. Blueberries' antibiotic properties block bacteria entry in the urinary tract which in turn, prevents infections.

Because they are delicious, you shouldn't have any problem eating blueberries by themselves. You can also add them to fruit salad, or to your favorite smoothie recipe.

Cranberries

Cranberries are excellent in preventing urinary tract infections. The antibacterial property of cranberries also aid in the elimination different toxins from the body. They are also loaded with anti-inflammatory nutrients. Eating cranberries will give you much needed cardiovascular support. They can boost your immune system and promote digestive health.

Goji Berries

Goji berries are very nutrient-dense. Eating Goji berries can naturally boost your beta-carotene and vitamin C levels. As you may know, vitamin C is very much helpful in detoxing, while beta-carotene can help improve your liver function.

Grapefruit

Grapefruit is a great source of antioxidants and vitamin C. It also helps increase the natural cleansing ability of the liver. Grapefruit juice for instance, can enhance the healthy production of enzymes which are essential for liver detoxification. Such enzymes have the ability to eliminate carcinogens and other toxic substances.

Lemon and Lime

Rich in Vitamin C, lemons and limes assist in toxic substances synthesis. Such makes them easily absorbed by water. With a glass of lemon or lime juice, especially in the morning, your liver receives proper stimulation.

Pineapple

This is another fruit worthy of mention when it comes to cleansing. Rich in the digestive enzyme bromelain, pineapple is quite effective in improving digestion and cleansing the colon.

Pomegranate

Loaded with anthocyanins, pomegranate provides the body with a serious antioxidant boost. Anthocyanins are believed to prevent inflammation and DNA damage. It is also helpful in reducing a person's risk of diabetes, allergies, heart disease and cancer. These antioxidants also have the ability to slow skin aging by reducing the weakening of elastin fibers and collagen.

Other Recommended Foods for Detox and Weight Loss

As a general rule in Fruit detox, you can take any fruits in their raw form. While your diet should consist mainly of fruits, you may also include vegetables and spices.

Beets and Carrots

These are both useful in the enhancement of the liver function. They are rich in plant-flavonoids as well as beta carotene which is known to cause liver stimulation.

Leafy Green Vegetables

You can eat your leafy greens raw, juiced, or cooked. They are rich in plant chlorophylls that filter environmental toxins and prevent them from entering the blood stream. They can effectively neutralize chemicals, heavy metals and pesticides. As a result, leafy green vegetables are quite effective in giving the liver a much needed protective mechanism. Dandelion greens, arugula, bitter gourd, spinach, chicoy and mustard greens can also help the liver with bile production and improve its flow.

Olive Oil

Used in moderation, olive oil can greatly benefit the liver. It provides a lipid base that is capable of capturing harmful toxins. Because of this, the burden of filtration and the usual workload of the liver may be eased.

Cruciferous Vegetables

Cauliflower and broccoli are helpful in increasing the level of glucosinolate within the body. This aids in the production of enzymes by the liver. These enzymes have the capability to get rid of toxins and carcinogens. This way, you may be able to lower your risk of developing cancer and other medical conditions.

Walnuts

Walnuts which contain arginine, an amino acid, are helpful to the liver, specifically with neutralizing ammonia. They are also rich in omega-3 fatty acids and glutathione, thus further enhancing the cleansing ability of the organ.

Cabbage

Cabbage is also capable of stimulating the production of liver detoxifying enzymes which make the liver more capable of removing toxins.

There are other foods that may prove to be helpful in cleansing, including asparagus, broccoli, brussel sprouts, artichoke and kale among others. Consuming these foods can absolutely help with your aim to boost liver function. As a result, you will be able to more effectively digest fat and successfully shed off the extra pounds.

Chapter 3:
How to Get Started with and Follow the Program

The rule of a fruit detox diet is simple. That is to eat only fruits and vegetables, preferably in their raw form. But how exactly do you start with this detox program? Here's how.

Avoid what is not good.

The first step to cleansing is eliminating the things that are known causes of stress to the liver. Such things can also lower your metabolic rate. These foods include artificial sweeteners, sugar, trans-fats, processed foods, soda, caffeine, over the counter drugs, and refined carbohydrates such as milk, gluten, white rice, cheese and soy protein isolates among others.

Alcohol is one of the major contributors of toxins in the body and it can directly take a toll on the liver. In which case, it is strongly recommended that you eliminate alcohol from your consumption. Drinking too much alcohol can also lead to cirrhosis, where the liver becomes so damaged that it's unable to filter toxins.

By minimizing your alcohol intake whether in the form of wine, beer, vodka, gin or rum, you can give your liver a rest. There are certain conditions that you can develop as a result of alcohol consumption, but the damage may often be reversed if you make an effort to quit drinking. Other food and elements that are known enemies to the liver are chemical additives, tap water, smoke, aerosol sprays, some medications, paints, black pepper, recycled or stale air, and insecticides or pesticides.

Start by consuming more fruits.

Make sure to incorporate fruits in your diet. Replace your sugary desserts with a serving of fruit. Have fruits for desserts daily, and after every meal. Instead of your usual snacks, eat fruits instead.

Go for foods that are good for the organs.

It is strongly suggested that you nourish your body with foods that offer liver support. Take note of the list of recommended foods for detox from the previous chapter.

In addition to fruit consumption, do not forget your cruciferous vegetables. Make sure to eat at least a cup's serving daily. You can have broccoli, cauliflower, cabbage and Brussel-sprouts. Green leafy vegetables must be included as well. Herbs such as dandelion greens, kale, chard, parsley, collards, watercress, mustard greens and the like are also helpful when detoxing.

Start your day with a glass of orange juice, or juice from a lemon or lime. Half a cup of onions, a clove of garlic and a quarter of a cup of daikon radish with cooked artichoke hearts and celery stalks can further help with liver cleansing. Also, half a cup of asparagus, a cup of beets, one or two teaspoons of yeast flakes, twenty grams of whey protein and one or two cups of dandelion tea are good for relieving and stimulating the liver function as well.

Take the time to prepare for the fruit cleanse.

Do not just jump into a detox right away. It's important to ease into this detox diet. You can do so by consuming foods that can offer support. For instance, start by adding a cup of berries, raw apple, pear or carrot, and two to three tablespoons of flaxseeds to your diet, while eliminating things like alcohol and processed foods.

A sudden change in your diet can only worsen side effects. Take your time in preparing. Remember that this detox diet is restrictive. You have to be prepared physically, mentally and emotionally.

Day One of Fruit Detox: What You Should Be Having

Prepare a sugar-free protein shake. Start your day by drinking 6 ounces of protein shake, and make sure you get yourself a serving every two hours to make a total of 5 drinks during the day. For dinner, you can have grilled lean chicken with a leafy green vegetable salad on the side and lemon or olive oil dressing.

Alternatively, for your protein consumption, you can take grass fed and low fat beef. Skinless chicken and turkey, lamb, fish and eggs rich in omega-3 are also recommended.

You need your dose of protein. The consumption of protein shall help reduce your cravings and hunger pangs. Your first day of diet is meant to prepare your body metabolism for the next few days. At the same time, it serves the purpose of excess fat burning.

Day Two of Fruit Detox: What You Should Be Having

On your second day, the protein shakes must be replaced with fruit. That means you should start your day by eating a serving of fresh fruit, and you have to make sure that you eat fresh fruits every two hours to prevent hunger. In total, you should have 5 servings of fruits during the day. You can take your pick from the list of recommended fruits in the previous chapter. Snacking in the evening is not allowed.

As for dinner, you may have a green salad with the best vegetables for detox. Season the salad with herbs and spices to further help boost weight loss. Pair your salad with half of an avocado. Also have a protein shake with dinner.

Day Three of Fruit Detox: What You Should Be Having

You can follow the same guidelines for the second day of detox. Choose fruits that are specifically rich in detoxifying properties. As much as possible, you should have fresh and organic produce.

Avoid canned and preserved fruits. Frozen and dried fruits are okay but ideally you should have your fruits fresh. If you get tired of eating whole fruits, you are allowed to juice them too.

The same applies for vegetables. For the salad, you can have any vegetable as long as you steer clear from the starchy ones like potatoes.

The cleansing process starts at day one. Days two and three are meant to further cleanse and rejuvenate your system. Fruits and vegetables are very much helpful in the process, with their nutrients, vitamins, minerals, water and fiber content.

Drink plenty of water.

As you go through the diet, make sure to have plenty of water. Water helps to relieve hunger. Moreover, during detox, your body is at a higher risk of dehydration so make sure to supplement lost water from your body. Furthermore, drinking plenty of water can help aid the cleansing process.

Drinking lots of fluids will also help in preparing your body for the cleansing process much better.

Get much needed fluids from other sources.

If you get tired of water, you can try a fruit infused water. You may also juice your fruits and vegetables. Try cranberry juice or lemon juice. Juice from a lemon or lime can also help with invigorating the liver. It can further help with dissolving fat so that it becomes much easier to flush out of your system.

To make a delicious cranberry juice that is best for cleansing, try this. Take eight ounces of the juice and mix it in filtered water that measures fifty six ounces. Boil the mixture lightly and add nutmeg, half a teaspoon of ground cinnamon, and a quarter teaspoon of ginger.

Simmer this combination for twenty minutes. After which, you can add a quarter cup of lemon juice, three quarters of a cup of orange juice, and some stevia.

As soon as you wake up, take two teaspoons of powdered psyllium husk mixed in water. You can also take two or three tablespoons of milled flaxseed in juice or water.

You can continue consuming cranberry juice, at least a cup a day, after the three day cleanse.

Ease out of the diet slowly.

After your third day, do not just go back to eating unhealthy foods again. Remember how tough it was to go through the detox. By this time, your body has rid itself of plenty of toxins. You will most likely lose weight as well. And to continue losing weight, avoid foods that make you fat. Steer clear from processed and sugary stuff. Swear them off.

On your fourth day, have a protein shake in the morning. A fruit smoothie will also do. Proceed to lunch with a fruit salad bowl and another protein shake. For the evening, have a protein dose in the form of lean meat, fish or chicken mixed with a green salad.

Reintroduce more foods back into your diet slowly. This way, you can avoid gastrointestinal problems. You know when your body is ready so listen to it well.

Keep avoiding foods that may stress the liver.

In the succeeding three days following the detox, it is important that you keep abstaining from the kinds of food that cause strain to your liver. At the same time, continue consuming those that provide support to this vital organ.

You can use the same foods that you have taken in preparation of the cleansing diet, and continue to drink plenty of water. In addition, you may also include a probiotic food. You can take a cup of yogurt for instance.

Chapter 4:
Juicing Guidelines on Fruit Detox Diet

Juices are also allowed in the fruit detox diet. Again, they should consist mainly of fruits and other healthy vegetables. For vegetables, cucumbers, carrots, tomatoes, beets, zucchini, romaine lettuce, squash, sprouts, cabbage and celery are recommended. Freshly squeezed juices from grapes, apples, and melons are also advised.

When juicing fruits and vegetables, it's important that you peel them first, especially those that may have been sprayed on or waxed. Cucumbers for instance are often waxed. Underground vegetables do not require peeling. Scrubbing and rinsing them may be enough.

It's important that you drink the juice as soon as you are done preparing it. It is from fresh juice that you can obtain a huge amount of vitamins and food enzymes. However, these may be lost if you let it sit for a long time.

How much do you need?

You can actually have as much as you want. It's difficult to overdo it, after all, it's good food. For juices, you can have an average of three or four glasses a day with each measuring eight ounces. You can have them before or in between meals.

The more you drink, the more you excrete. You may notice that you urinate often and you have increased bowel movements. That's just your body's natural reaction.

Which juices are good for you?

You can refer to the suggested food list and pick whatever appeals to you. You can even combine fruits and vegetable together. Below are some of the most popular choices.

Carrot Juice

Carrots are Vitamin A enriched. It's sweet tasting and because it's non-toxic, you are free to have as much as you want.

Before you juice the carrots, make sure you brush them. You may peel them, but it's not necessary since this is an underground vegetable. Using a tough brush to clean its outer covering is enough.

Celery juice

Do not juice celery alone. You may add it in combination with other fruits and vegetables. Consuming too much celery juice is not advised. That is because they are a little high in sodium.

You can add them to juice for flavor. And make sure you use the leaves because they offer the greatest number of health benefits.

Cucumber juice

Another tasty juice drink comes from cucumber. It has a similar taste to watermelon. Before you juice cucumber, make sure you peel the skin off. They're often waxed and so washing isn't enough.

Cabbage juice

Cabbage juice was used to treat peptic ulcers in the 1950's. Since that time, cabbage juice has gained recognition and is now used for the treatment of gastrointestinal disorders. For instance, spastic colon, chronic constipation, colitis, indigestion and other conditions respond well to the nutritional content cabbage juice has to offer. It is interesting to note that cabbage along with broccoli is recognized for their cancer fighting abilities.

Zucchini squash

This may seem like a strange combination but it can actually taste good. It is a good way to take a short break from high fiber juices and vegetables.

Romaine lettuce

This juice is rich in chlorophyll and minerals. It may take some time for you to get used to the taste but it does your body a lot of good.

Beet juice

Peel the beets before you attempt to juice them. It is considered as a blood builder. And although they have a bitter tasting skin, the inside is actually quite tasty and sweet. It does have a strong color though which can stain whatever it comes into contact with including your bowels.

Tomato juice

Pick the ripe and red kind of tomatoes. They taste fine and they are also quite easy to juice.

Leafy green vegetables can be juiced as well. Some good examples include beet greens, parsley, chard, kale, spinach and dandelion greens. Cruciferous vegetables including cabbage, broccoli and Brussel sprouts are also good for health, as well as root vegetables like sweet potatoes and beets. Cranberries, peaches, strawberries, watermelon, pineapple and citrus fruits also make healthy options.

In addition to fruits and vegetables, herbs may be added for flavor. Spearmint, yucca, fennel, peppermint, ginger, basil, garlic and the like can be juiced, not just for better taste, but they also offer health benefits. Bean sprouts and wheatgrass will also make a good addition to your juice as well as aloe Vera gel which is often taken for arthritis treatment.

Chapter 5:
What to Expect on a Fruit Detox Diet

This detox diet plan works by eliminating toxins from the body. It is also intended to jump start weight loss. The fruit cleanse diet in particular, created by Jay Robb lasts for three days. This particular cleansing diet features nutritious foods, so there are only a few side effects that dieters may experience. And in comparison to other crash diets, the side effects from a fruit detox are not usually severe and not generally common.

Who can benefit from this detox diet?

Healthy people and those in good physical condition can benefit enormously from Fruit Detox. But there are certain individuals who are not suited for this kind of detoxification method. For instance, pregnant and nursing women should not go through this cleansing diet. It is also not advisable for children.

If you have diabetes, anorexia, hypoglycemia, epilepsy, asthma, gout, kidney or liver disease, anemia, ulcerative colitis, impaired immune system, active infections and terminal illness, this cleansing diet is prohibited. Individuals who are way below their recommended weight are also discouraged from this diet and so are people who have recently gone surgery.

Fruit Detox can be beneficial but it is advised to be performed only for about three to four days. Anything beyond this time frame should be medically supervised. The longer you perform the diet, the lesser nutrition enters your body. And such can cause deficiencies which will do more harm than good to your overall health.

During the fruit detox program, people normally feel fatigued, dizzy and nauseated. Blood pressure may decrease and vomiting may be experienced. These side effects should go away by themselves as the fasting comes to a close. However, if they reach a certain level where the side effects are no longer tolerable, it is in your best interest to stop the fasting and consult a doctor immediately. Other usual side effects include headaches, increased body odor, bad breath, constipation and acne.

The Most Common Side Effects

Similar to other detox diets, individuals who apply the fruit detox may experience headaches. Fatigue is also common as well as dehydration. This is why dieters are stroungly encouraged to drink plenty of water. Drinking a sufficient amount of water also enhances the impact of detoxification further.

Gastrointestinal Issues

Another common side effect is gastrointestinal issues. And this is especially true for people who have been eating an unhealthy diet. The dieter's system attempts to adjust to the new diet and as a result, gastrointestinal problems may occur.

Among such gastrointestinal issues include abdominal pain, nausea, diarrhea and bloating. The severity of these side effects varies from one individual to another.

Other Things to Expect

Like other restrictive diets, this cleansing program may cause a disruption in the blood sugar levels. It also possibly reduces electrolytes in the body. During this diet, your sodium and potassium levels may be compromised which means hunger and food cravings are quite common. In addition, shakiness and muscle weakness may also be experienced.

With all these effects and restrictions in mind, not all individuals are advised to follow the program. Specifically, pregnant and breastfeeding women should steer clear from this diet and all other kinds of restrictive diets for that matter. People with diabetes, kidney and heart diseases are also advised to avoid this detox diet. Elderly people and children should be discouraged from undertaking it as well.

If you are planning to lose weight or to improve overall health with the help of this detox plan, it is wise to consult your doctor first, a nutritionist or a dietitian. That way, you can maximize the effects of this detox diet without compromising your overall health.

Conclusion

Thank you again for downloading this book!

I hope this book was able to help you learn more about detoxing, and how you can do one to improve your health.

Remember to first decide if this detox diet is suitable for you, before giving it a go!

The next step is to put this information to use, and begin your own fruit detox!

Finally, if you enjoyed this book, please take the time to share your thoughts and post a review on Amazon. It'd be greatly appreciated!

Thank you and good luck!

www.ingramcontent.com/pod-product-compliance
Lightning Source LLC
LaVergne TN
LVHW021750060526
838200LV00052B/3571